You Can Get There From Here

Hiking Hunterdon County Trails

Happy Trails!
Alice Oldford
Sue Dziamara

Alice Oldford and Sue Dziamara

iUniverse, Inc.
New York Bloomington

You Can Get There From Here
Hiking Hunterdon County Trails

Photos courtesy of Jim Graham

iUniverse books may be ordered through booksellers or by contacting:

iUniverse
1663 Liberty Drive
Bloomington, IN 47403
www.iuniverse.com
1-800-Authors (1-800-288-4677)

Because of the dynamic nature of the Internet, any Web addresses or links contained in this book may have changed since publication and may no longer be valid.

ISBN: 978-1-4401-5859-9 (sc)
ISBN: 978-1-4401-5860-5 (ebk)

Printed in the United States of America

iUniverse rev. date: 8/4/2009

Contents

Acknowledgements vii

Introduction   What to Expect and Preparing for Your Hike 1

Chapter 1   Charlestown Reservation, Bethlehem Township 3

Chapter 2   Jugtown Mountain Nature Preserve, Bethlehem
             Township 7

Chapter 3   Echo Hill Environmental Education Area, Clinton
             Township 9

Chapter 4   Hunterdon County Arboretum, Clinton Township. .13

Chapter 5   Sunnyside Picnic Area and Awossogame Grove,
             Clinton Township. 17

Chapter 6   Cushetunk Mountain Nature Preserve, Clinton and
             Readington Townships 21

Chapter 7   Round Valley Reservoir, Clinton and Readington
             Townships. 25

Chapter 8   Winter Wanderings, Town of Clinton. 29

Chapter 9   Landsdown Trail, Franklin Township and Town of
             Clinton. 33

Chapter 10   Deerpath Park and Round Mountain Section,
             Readington Township. 37

Chapter 11   Hoffman Park, Union Township. 41

Chapter 12   The Columbia Trail, High Bridge and Califon
             Boroughs, Clinton and Lebanon Townships 45

Chapter 13   Crystal Springs Section of the Teetertown Preserve,
             Lebanon Township 49

Chapter 14   Miquin Woods, Lebanon Township 53

Chapter 15   Musconetcong River Reservation: Point Mountain
             Section, Lebanon Township 57

Chapter 16   Teetertown Preserve, including Mountain Farm
             Section, Lebanon Township 61

Chapter 17   Voorhees State Park, Lebanon Township. 65

Chapter 18   Cold Brook Reserve, Tewksbury Township 69

Chapter 19   End of the Trail. 73

About the Authors. 75

Acknowledgements

Special thanks to Jim Graham, friend/walking partner/photographer for his many hours spent exploring the trails.

Heartfelt appreciation to Alison Oldford for her design, editorial and web expertise and guidance and to Evan Oldford for his words of wisdom.

Thanks to our editor, Barbara Benjamin, for her insights and encouragement.

Thanks to Josie Agosto for helping format the photos.

Thanks to Douglas Martin for sharing his knowledge about the history of the Bethlehem Baptist Church.

Thanks to John Hoinowski for explaining the hunter's perspective on the parks.

Thanks to our families and friends for their support and encouragement.

What to Expect and Preparing for Your Hike

Hunterdon County's rural character is an oasis in western central New Jersey, the most densely populated state in the United States. Part of the Skylands Region, Hunterdon County is bounded on the west by the Delaware River with a view of Pennsylvania. Farm fields, forests, hills, wildlife, and two reservoirs as well as historic homes, farms, and estates describe Hunterdon County. The County is home to parks and trails offering outdoor opportunities to people of all ages.

Living in a bedroom community, many of Hunterdon's residents commute east more than two hours a day to work in New York City. Their time is precious, but they crave the benefits of living in beautiful and serene Hunterdon County.

Sue and I met while serving on the Clinton Township Planning Board and began to explore the trails for the exercise, the serenity, and the joy of being outside. Sharing our excitement with friends and colleagues, we discovered that many people had no idea what Hunterdon County trails have to offer.

It occurred to us to share the wealth as we have experienced it. Each season brings a new perspective. We thought it would be helpful to let people know what they can expect to encounter.

The degree of difficulty ratings that we use throughout this book are subjective, which are the following:

Easy - Suitable for folks with good sneakers who spend more time in the work environment than exercising. Easy works, too, for families with children approximately 8 years of age and younger. Sore muscles on your return to work on Monday should not be an issue.

Moderate - Shoes sturdier than sneakers are recommended, as well as a water bottle. If you are bringing the family, we believe that children 9-12 years could appreciate these trails. There is likely to be some rolling terrain. Trails in the moderate category could cause you to break a sweat and become aware that your muscles had spent a sedentary week. If you do get in some walking or time in the gym during the week, moderate trails will be fun.

Challenging - Let's say you need a challenge, either for body or mind, go for trails that we classify as challenging. Be sure that you have hiking or sturdy shoes, water, and perhaps a snack. You will encounter rocks, even boulders, and some steep hills. Children ages 13 and older should be able to handle these trails.

For any of the categories, by all means bring your camera. Seasonally there are all sorts of things of interest that you might want to share, from goslings in spring to glistening virgin snow in winter.

The trails are listed here according to municipality for ease in your choice of where to go on an outing.

Enjoy the trails year round, and we encourage you to do some exploring on your own.

Charlestown Reservation

Desire is the starting point of all achievement, not a hope, not a wish, but a keen pulsating desire which transcends everything.
-- Napolean Hill

Difficulty Rating: Moderate
Distance: 2 miles
Sun/Shade: Mostly shade
Location: Bethlehem Township
Highlights: Views, wildlife
Restrooms: No
Parking: Gravel
Hunting: Yes
Directions:

> From the junction with Route 78, go north on Route 31 approximately 6 miles. Make a left at the traffic light at Glen Manor Road. Proceed to the end of the road. Turn left onto Black Brook Road and make the first right onto Charlestown Lane. At the end of Charlestown Lane, make a left onto Route 635. The entrance to Charlestown Reservation is on the right.

Now designated as a conservation area, this property of 215 acres was originally a tree farm. Later it was used for agricultural crops, such as corn and wheat, and an apple orchard was also established. This gives a sense of the diversity that you will encounter.

Long pants and hiking shoes are in order. The difficulty rating for this hike is moderate, starting with a climb from the trailhead on Charlestown Road. This trail is rugged enough that we would not recommend taking small children (those younger than 5 years). Plan to spend a couple of hours to fully appreciate the trail.

You will find an old field road and rock hedgerow as you discover this park. You could be treated to a view of a variety of wildlife, including the grey fox. A wide range of woodland bird species inhabits the park as well. Watch for tufted titmice and black-capped chickadees. Look up to see red-tailed hawks and turkey vultures.

To control the deer population, hunting is permitted in the park with a special hunting license issued by the County Parks Department in addition to a New Jersey Division of Fish and Wildlife license. Six permits are issued for the 215 huntable acres. Hunting is not permitted on Sundays. For complete details, please see the Hunterdon County Department of Parks and Recreation website, www.co.hunterdon.nj.us.

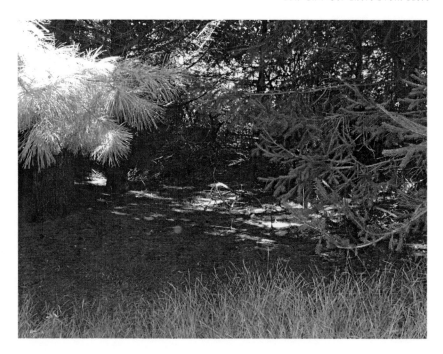

Charlestown - deer watching us

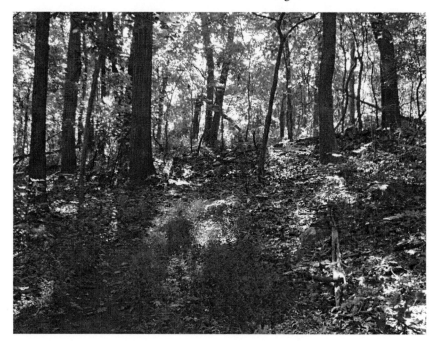

Charlestown - terrain

Jugtown Mountain Nature Preserve

Focus on remedies, not faults.
-- Jack Nicklaus

Difficulty Rating: Moderate
Distance: 2.17 miles
Sun/Shade: Shade
Location: Bethlehem Township
Restrooms: No
Highlights: Rocks, mining history, views
Parking: Dirt
Hunting: Yes
Directions:
>From Route 78, go West to Exit 11. Proceed on Route 173 West for about 2 miles. Turn right onto Mine Road. The entrance to the park is on the left just beyond the Bethlehem Township Municipal Building.

It is shady and cool in the Jugtown Mountain Nature Preserve, and the hiking difficulty is moderate. You can hike the entire trail in one hour. Hiking boots and long pants are recommended.

Although we do not recommend this trail for young children, we think it could be interesting to somewhat older children, say 8 and older, because of the interesting rocks, critters, and perhaps the history. In some areas, depending on the time of year, there are locations where you can overlook the Musconetcong Watershed.

Wildlife habitat is abundant. See spotted salamanders and wood frogs that inhabit numerous vernal pools. The stone walls and rock fields provide shelter to snakes and rodents.

Although its name identifies with moonshiners, who hid their jugs on rock ledges to avoid the authorities during prohibition, the history of the 153-acre preserve is in mining. The Swayze mine, which was located in the Preserve, was one of the top three producers of magnetic ore. At its peak, it produced 10,000 tons of ore annually before closing in 1889. You can still see remnants of mining activities, including rock pits and ore dumps.

To control the deer population, hunting is allowed in the park with a special hunting license issued by the County Parks Department in addition to a New Jersey Division of Fish and Wildlife license. Eight permits are issued for the 211 huntable acres within this preserve. Hunting is not permitted on Sundays. For complete details, please see the Hunterdon County Department of Parks and Recreation website, www.co.hunterdon.nj.us.

Echo Hill Environmental Education Area

Your attitude is the control center of your life.
-- Angela C. Gonzalez and Richard W. Cronen

Difficulty Rating: Easy
Distance: 1.25 miles
Sun/Shade: Sun and shade
Location: Clinton Township
Highlights: Multi-use, water, wildlife
Restrooms: Yes
Parking: Paved
Hunting: Yes, limited hours
Directions:
>Take Route 31 to Stanton Station Road. Travel 0.4 mile to Lilac Drive. At Lilac Drive turn right and proceed another 0.4 mile. The entrance to the Echo Hill Environmental Education park will be on the right. Follow the sign to the main parking area.

As a farm established in 1836, Echo Hill was comprised of a stone house, a barn, chicken coops, and a peach orchard. Today the stone farm house headquarters the South Branch Watershed Association. In 1936, Robert and Hermia Lechner purchased the property and established a summer camp for children. Then in 1939, the Civilian Conservation Corps (CCC) was instrumental in converting the farm to a summer camp. True to its name, the CCC reused buildings or materials from the buildings, and 200,000 evergreen seedlings replaced the peach orchard. The County acquired the property in 1973 and continues its teaching traditions through various programs.

The Echo Hill Environmental Education park offers many options for family use, including hiking trails, a playground and picnic area adjacent to the parking lot, plus organized group camping by reservation. Catch-and-release fishing is allowed in the pond. The main activity center provides meeting rooms and kitchenette available by reservation.

Hikers can enjoy easy–to-moderate hiking through various habitats. Consider a perimeter hike through varied terrain with open fields and woods, which can be done in less than one hour. The trails are suitable for family use, but long pants are recommended. You will enjoy a great view of the Prescott Brook. When the water level allows, you will be able to cross the Prescott Brook and walk through the tunnel across Route 31 to the Hunterdon County Arboretum. The stream crossing is well marked.

If you enjoy bird watching, you will find that feeding stations have been installed to attract songbirds, and a seasonal bird blind is available on a bluff overlooking the pond. A summertime bonus is wild raspberry picking adjacent to the parking lot.

Archery and winter bow hunting (September–November and January–February) are allowed in the park with a special hunting license issued by the County Parks Department in addition to a New Jersey Division of Fish and Game Wildlife license. Three permits are issued for the 90 huntable acres. Hunting is not permitted from 10 a.m. to 2 p.m. daily. For complete details, please see the Hunterdon County Department of Parks and Recreation website, www.co.hunterdon.nj.us.

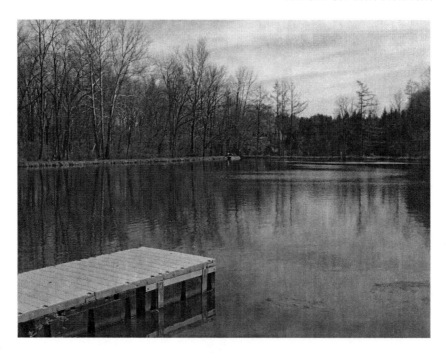

Echo Hill - pond

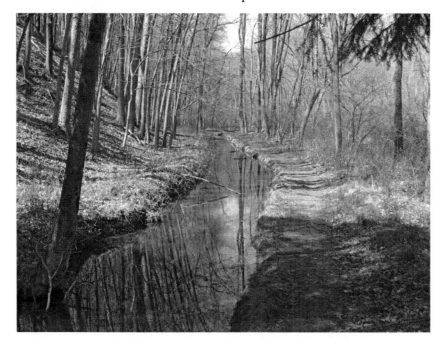

Echo Hill - spillway

Hunterdon County Arboretum

No matter how good you get, you can always get better and that's the exciting part.
-- Tiger Woods

Difficulty Rating: Easy
Distance: 1.1 miles
Sun/Shade: Sun and shade
Location: Clinton Township
Highlights: Education, gardens
Restrooms: Yes, in the building when it is open
Parking: Gravel
Hunting: Yes, limited hours
Directions:

> The Arboretum is located on Route 31N in Clinton Township, 5 miles south of Clinton and 5 miles north of Flemington.

If you are looking for a family outing, the Arboretum has it all. Boasting shade, some meadows and wetlands, plus a pond, this is a great four-season opportunity. The winter bonus is cross-country skiing.

The Hunterdon County Department of Parks and Recreation maintains its office at this 73-acre site, formerly a commercial nursery, and each season they seem to conceive a new attraction. The arboretum is the Park System's showcase, and they sponsor various educational programs and recreational opportunities throughout the year.

The Outer Loop path is 1.1 miles, with the Discovery, Memorial, and Two-Line trails crisscrossing. If you are feeling adventurous, follow the tunnel under Route 31; and if the river is low enough, you can cross to the Echo Hill Park.

The Arboretum is a fun place to explore – truly offering something for everyone. And when you're ready for a break, choose your picnic table. A visit to the reconstructed gazebo is a treat, and you can be transported to a quieter, gentler place meandering on the brick path through the perennial gardens.

For the kids, there is a castle with telescopes to keep watch. Visit the alphabet herb garden, and enjoy the vegetable garden in summer.

For the adults wishing for a stress-free place for contemplation, they can rest on a bench in the garden that contains a fountain.

Archery and winter bow hunting is allowed in the park September–November and January–February with a special hunting license issued by the County Parks Department in addition to a New Jersey Division of Fish and Wildlife license. Three permits are issued for the huntable 73 acres, with no hunting permitted from 10 a.m. to 2 p.m. daily. For complete details, please see the Hunterdon County Department of Parks and Recreation website, www.co.hunterdon.nj.us.

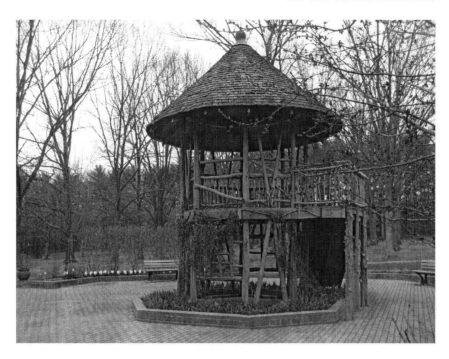

Arboretum - gazebo

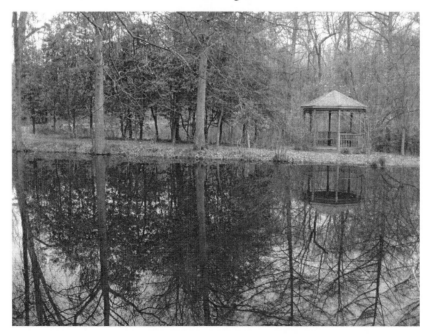

Arboretum - pond

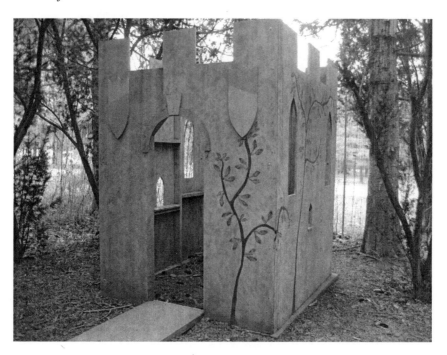

Arboretum - castle on wizard's walk

Sunnyside Picnic Area and Awossogame Grove

Let us run with perseverance the race that is set before us.
-- RSV Hebrews 12:1

Difficulty Rating: Easy
Distance: 1.15 miles
Sun/Shade: Mostly shade
Location: Clinton Township
Highlights: River, 911 Memorial
Restrooms: No
Parking: Gravel
Hunting: No
Directions from the Clinton Area:

>Take Route 31S approximately 5 miles from Route 78 to the traffic light for Payne Road. Turn right onto Payne Road and proceed to the end. Turn left onto Lilac Drive and proceed for a little more than a mile. Turn right at Kiceniuk Road. After crossing the railroad tracks, Kiceniuk Road bears to the right. Continue along Kiceniuk. The parking lot is on the left just before the bridge.

Part of the South Branch Reservation that helps preserve the watershed of the South Branch of the Raritan River, the trail is suited to an easy summer walk along the river. The walk is short, not more than 30 minutes. Four picnic sites make it ideal for a family picnic. Access is provided to the river for fishing or launching a canoe.

Sunnyside park is also the site of Awossogame Grove, a memorial to the Hunterdon County victims of 9/11. The Hunterdon County Freeholders selected this location because it is close both to the heart of Hunterdon and to the river.

The Lenni Lenape Indians camped in this area, and Awossogame is translated from their native tongue to mean "place out of sight," construed as heaven. Twenty trees in all were planted to remember the Hunterdon victims of the terrorist attack. Five arrowwood vibernum bushes were planted to signify the five points of the Pentagon. The Lenni Lenape used arrowwood vibernum to make arrows. When a tribe member died, they would shoot an arrow and bury the tribe member where the arrow landed.

A gneiss rock found in Lebanon Township was placed at the memorial site with a memorial plaque mounted on the rock. The site was dedicated on September 11, 2006.

In addition to the rich heritage of Native Americans in the area, the home of Jacob Gearhart, one of the procurers of boats for George Washington's crossing of the Delaware on Christmas Day, is located along the River Road. This is a stone house identified with a marker as the home of Jacob Gearhart.

No hunting is permitted in this park.

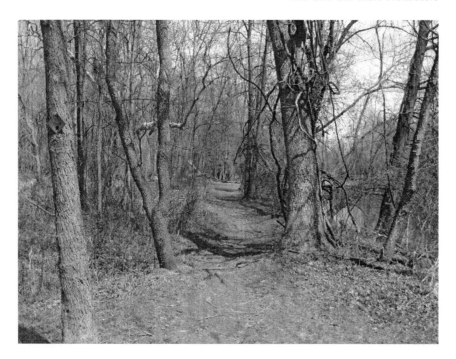

Sunnyside - view of trail

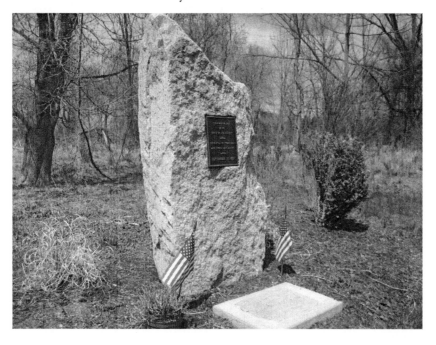

Sunnyside - 911 Memorial

Cushetunk Mountain Nature Preserve

If you can find a path with no obstacles, it probably doesn't lead anywhere.
--Frank A. Clark

Difficulty Rating: Challenging
Distance: 3.17 miles
Sun/Shade: Mostly shade
Location: Clinton Township, Readington Township
Highlights: Views, rocks, solitude
Restrooms: No
Parking: Dirt and gravel
Hunting: Yes
Directions:

> From Clinton, take Route 22 east. Turn right at Route 629, also known as the Round Valley Access Road. Proceed 1.4 miles and turn left at the Boat Launch Ramp. Follow this road for another 1.4 miles to Old Mountain Road. Turn right and travel 1.5 miles. Parking for the park is just before the railroad tracks on the right.

As a result of the steep inclines, the Cushetunk Mountain trail, adjacent to Round Valley Reservoir, is definitely not for the faint of heart. Long pants are in order and hiking shoes recommended. Do not forget your water, and chances are that you would be glad to have along an energy bar.

The mountains were formed by volcanic activity more than 160 million years ago. The Lenni Lenape Indians called the area *Cushetunk*, which means "place of hogs." You can almost envision the wild hogs traversing the narrow trails.

Although we've not seen them, we know that there is a pair of nesting eagles there, and we have heard the eaglets. The trail is closed from April 1 to August 1 to not disturb the eagles and their off-spring.

A great two-hour hike from the parking area starts where the trail is closed seasonally for the nesting eagles. The trail is well marked with white markers, and you will be heading upward. When reaching the top, you will be treated to a great view of the reservoir. Now proceed along the ridge trail, which is very rocky and dotted with rock outcroppings perfect for a break or a little personal meditation. The markers on this trail stop abruptly, which may present a dilemma whether to continue on or to turn back. If you feel a little adventurous, do go on. Keep the yellow Park System signs in sight, and you will encounter a trail (or path), which may or may not be marked where you pick it up. Head down the hill, and you will see white blazes painted on the trees. It is an easy walk back, which will probably make you smile after your earlier exertion. Just follow the power lines back to the parking area.

Perhaps you have only 30 minutes for a short hike or you want to introduce your children to this bit of County history where the walk isn't too taxing. Walk out from the parking area, following the power lines, until you reach the start of a trail. It is single track through the woods, fairly level, and not too long –about 30 minutes.

To control the deer population, hunting is allowed in the park with a special hunting license issued by the County Parks Department in addition to a New Jersey Division of Fish and Wildlife license. Twenty permits are issued for the 380 huntable acres. For complete details, please see the Hunterdon County Department of Parks and Recreation website, www.co.hunterdon. nj.us.

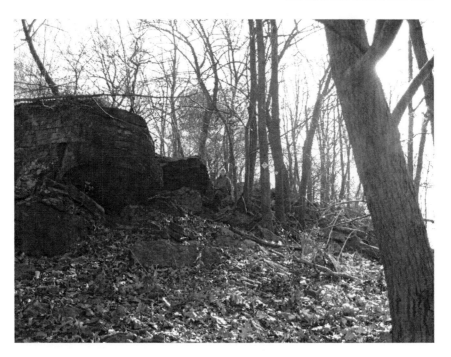

Cushetunk - ridge trail

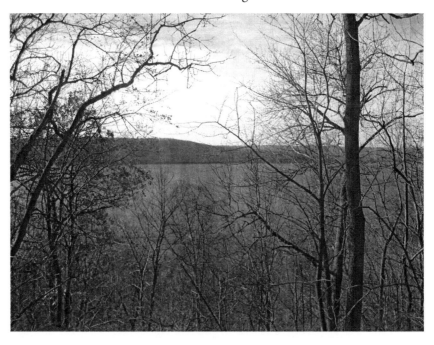

Cushetunk - view of Round Valley Reservoir

Round Valley Reservoir

The best and most beautiful things in the world cannot be seen or even touched.
They must be felt with the heart.
-- Helen Keller

Difficulty Rating: Easy to Challenging
Distance: 14 miles
Sun/Shade: Sun and shade
Location: Clinton Township
Highlights: Year-round, multi-use, reservoir, views, shade
Restrooms: Yes (open year round)
Parking: Paved
Hunting: Yes, waterfowl only
Directions:
> From Clinton, take Route 22 East. Turn right at Route 629,
> also known as the Round Valley Access Road. Proceed to the
> main entrance on the left.

Round Valley Reservoir, a state park, is a wonderful 2000+ acre year-round, multi-use family resource in our midst offering a variety of terrain and habitat. Fishing, swimming, boating, picnicking, and wilderness camping come to mind immediately. Winter offers sleigh riding, ice skating, and cross-country skiing for outdoor enthusiasts.

Round Valley was originally a volcano. In Revolutionary times, Round Valley was populated by several farm families. Round Valley was a safe haven because there was only one natural entrance. The state of New Jersey purchased the property in the 1950s with the goal of building a reservoir. During the 1960s, the houses were moved or demolished, and the valley was filled with water. As the deepest lake in New Jersey, Round Valley is approximately 180-feet deep with a capacity of 55 billion gallons. For a fascinating history of the reservoir, we suggest reading *Beneath These Waters,* written by Stephanie Stevens and published by the Hunterdon County Historical and Cultural Commission 2008.

Hiking is a year-round choice at the Round Valley Reservoir. Although there are many trail options to enjoy, no trail goes completely around the reservoir. Mountain biking and horseback riding are also permitted trail uses. Age-rated playground equipment is available in the beach area.

A day-use fee applies from Memorial Day through Labor Day.

To enjoy a moderate, one-hour hike, park in the south lot and pick up the trail beside the reservoir. This trail is less used, and you will negotiate some tall grass and brambles, so we recommend long pants. In addition to the reservoir, you will have a view of Cushetunk Mountain, where you might catch a glimpse of one of the nesting eagles. From this vantage point you will also see the dams. The trail leads you through the forest, up and down moderate hills, and you emerge near the boat launch parking area. Turn south and follow the trail through the forest and along the opposite side of the swimming area. You will emerge at the East Picnic area, and it is a short walk back to the south parking lot.

This is also a nice hike for a hot day or any time that you want to experience the tranquility and clarity of the water.

Hunting is limited to waterfowl. Hunting and fishing regulations are found at www.njfishandwildlife.com.

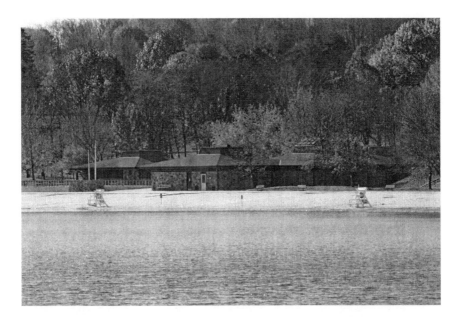

Round Valley - beach

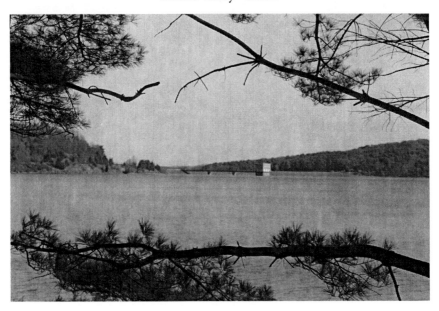

Round Valley - dam

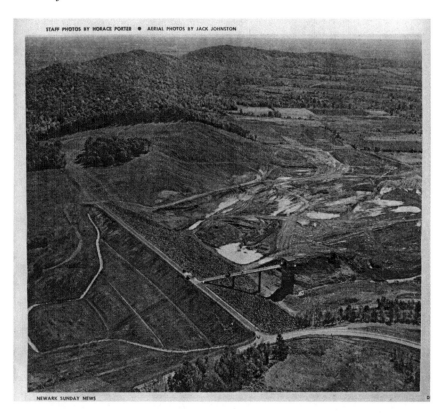

STAFF PHOTOS BY HORACE PORTER ● AERIAL PHOTOS BY JACK JOHNSTON

NEWARK SUNDAY NEWS

Round Valley - history

Winter Wanderings

The art of being wise is knowing what to overlook.
-- William James

Difficulty Rating: Easy
Distance: 3 miles
Sun/Shade: Mostly sun
Location: Town of Clinton
Highlights: Sidewalks, historic homes
Restrooms: Yes, at the library
Parking: Yes, paved, at the library
Hunting: No
Directions:

> From Route 78, take Route 173, also known as W. Main St., to Halstead Street. Follow Halstead Street to the North County Branch of the library located on the left.

It's wintertime, and there is snow and ice on the trails. It is very cold, and you really need to get outside. Here is an option.

Park at the North County library branch and head out on the sidewalk toward downtown Clinton. Walk through town on the sunny side of Main Street. Cross the bridge, and after looking at the Red Mill and dreaming about outside activities in the summer, continue on the sidewalk past the Clinton House on West Main Street.

Enjoy reminiscing about the historic homes and stay on Route 173 heading toward Route 78. Keep to the sidewalks and follow Lakeview Avenue up the hill and loop around on Kintner, then head back toward town the way you came. When you get back to town, stop for a bit of refreshment, if you like, and then take Lower Center Street. Cross Halstead Street and proceed on Center Street to New Street.

Alice Oldford and Sue Dziamara

Take New Street to East Main Street. Remember to stay on the sunny side. Follow to Halstead Street and back to the library.

Located on the South Branch of the Raritan River, the Town of Clinton was known as Hunt's Mill in the 1700's, named for the Hunts who built mills on the river. The red mill and the stone mill stand today offering visitors some insight into Clinton history. In 1929, the post office was established, and the town was named for New York Governor Dewitt Clinton.

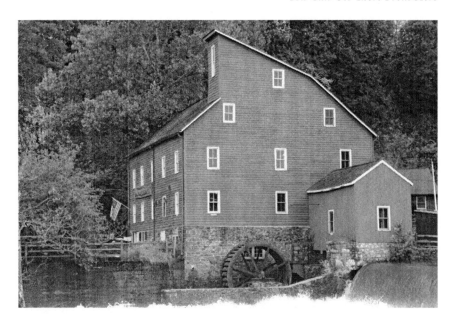

Clinton - red mill

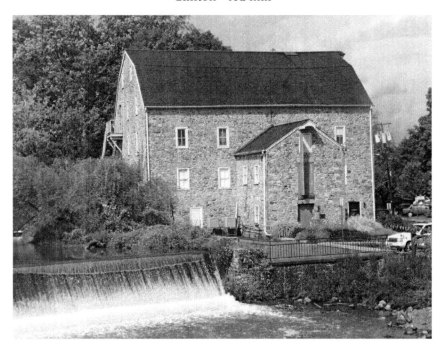

Clinton - stone mill

Landsdown Trail

If you can imagine it, you can achieve it; if you can dream it, you can become it.
-- William Arthur Ward

Difficulty Rating: Easy
Distance: 1.5 miles
Sun/Shade: Mostly shade
Location: Town of Clinton and Franklin Township
Highlights: Picturesque, multi-use, river
Restrooms: No
Parking: Park along Lower Landsdown Road or the public parking in Clinton
Hunting: No
Directions:
> In Clinton, the trailhead is located between Fox Lumber and the Clinton Global Ag.
> In Franklin, the trailhead is on Lower Landsdown Road over the railroad tracks beyond the Faith Chapel Wesleyan Church. Take Route 31 to Allerton Road, which becomes Wellington. Turn left on Leigh Street and right on Lower Landsdown to the trailhead.

In the late 1800s, the Landsdown Trail was a spur line for the Lehigh Valley Railroad. The line was used for passengers as well as moving freight to and from the Clinton Mill, formerly known as Mulligan's Mill. The old train station survives and is used by Fox Lumber as a showroom. The train station building won an award from the Hunterdon County Planning Board in 2007 for a tasteful rehabilitation.

Flat, safe, and picturesque, the Landsdown Trail was created from the railroad bed running along the South Branch of the Raritan River. Perfect for walking or biking in all seasons, this trail is suitable for the whole family. Cross-country skiing in the winter is a nice bonus.

Pick up the trail where the railroad tracks cross Lower Landsdown Road, walk 1.5 miles to Clinton, then enjoy lunch, coffee, or ice cream. Or start from Clinton, parking between Fox Lumber and Global Ag, and leave the highway noise behind.

Make an expedition by crossing to Landsdown Road and picking up the Capoolong Creek Trail. This is a well-shaded, flat path, sometimes wide and sometimes single track, running along the Capoolong Creek for 4 miles to Pittstown.

There is access to the South Branch of the Raritan River if fishing strikes your fancy.

No hunting is allowed in this park. However, there is hunting available in adjacent areas.

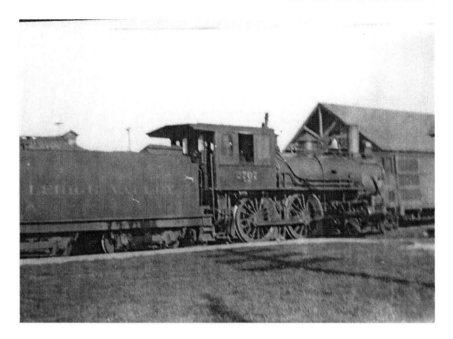

Laandsdown - train pulling into the station

Deerpath Park and Round Mountain Section

If you don't know where you're going, how will you get there?
-- Gregory McGuire

Difficulty Rating: Easy to Moderate
Distance: 5 miles
Sun/Shade: More sun, less shade
Location: Readington Township
Restrooms: Yes
Highlights: Recreational facilities, pond, rolling terrain
Parking: Paved
Hunting: Yes
Directions:
> From Clinton, take Route 31 south. Use the jughandle for West Woodschurch Road to cross over Route 31. Follow the signs for Deer Path Park and the YMCA. Continue past the YMCA entrance and turn right. The parking lot for the soccer fields is on the left-hand side of the driveway. The main parking lot for the park is located at the end of the driveway near the rest rooms.
>
> From Flemington, take Route 31 north. Turn right on West Woodschurch Road and follow the signs for Deerpath Park as above.

Deerpath Park was formerly used as a summer camp for children where the activities included swimming, boating, horseback riding, archery, and tennis. This park is now a wonderful multi-recreational use facility for the whole family. A 3-acre spring-fed pond, called Deerpath Pond, is easy to access. It is a catch-and-release pond suitable for children. Fish include bass, catfish, and sunfish.

Walk-in picnic sites with grills are available. In addition, pavilion facilities are available with reservations for groups of 25 or more. Reservations are made at the Hunterdon County Department of Parks and Recreation main office located at the Arboretum, (908) 782-1158.

Enjoy a little meditative time at the memorial gazebo and garden located along the pond. This is also a popular site for wedding photos. Reservations are required for photo opportunities.

Deerpath Park offers two soccer fields and a softball field, a one-mile fitness trail with twenty exercise stations, plus two miles of trails for walking or running. The trails are primarily mowed paths with rolling terrain. Remember the sunscreen because there is more sun than shade on the paths. The hiking is mostly easy. These trails also serve as the home course for the Hunterdon Central High School cross-country track team.

Deerpath Park is often the site for special events including performance camp, community festivals, and scout events, as well as the Summer Concert series. For a schedule of events, contact the Park Commission office.

Adjacent to Deerpath Park is the Round Mountain Section consisting of 236 acres with mowed paths and trails through the woods. The hiking in this section is moderate. In winter, cross-country skiing is a bonus.

The Round Mountain section was once used by the Lenni Lenape for encampments. Early European settlers cut timber for lumber and heating fuel and farmed the surrounding base of the mountain. The logging road has been incorporated into the trail system, and you can see the remnants of stone walls dividing farm fields.

The Round Mountain trail now connects to a Readington Township trail, identified as Peter Buell Trail. What a great way for a municipality to preserve land and create an active recreation opportunity.

To control the deer population, hunting is allowed in the park with a special license issued by the County Parks Department in addition to a New Jersey Division of Fish and Wildlife license. Four permits are issued for the 100 huntable acres. Hunting is not permitted on Sundays. For complete details, please see the Hunterdon County Department of Parks and Recreation website, www.co.hunterdon.nj.us.

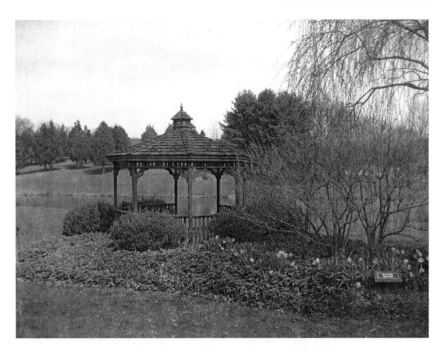

Deerpath - gazebo overlooking pond

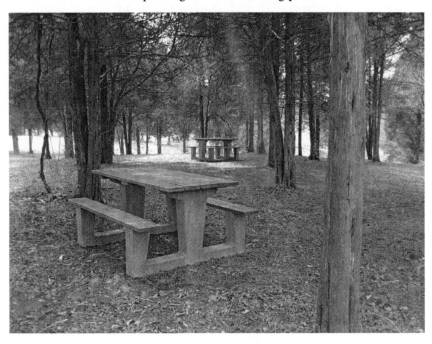

Deerpath - picnic area

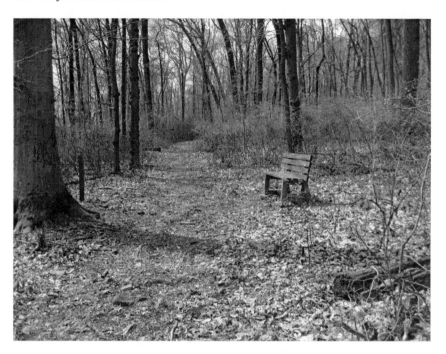

Round Mountain - bench along the trail

Hoffman Park

It's choice – not chance – that determines your destiny.
-- Jean Nidetch

Difficulty Rating: Easy
Distance: 3 miles
Sun/Shade: Shade, some sun
Location: Union Township
Highlights: Views, ponds, shade
Restrooms: Yes
Parking: Paved
Hunting: Yes
Directions:

From the East Clinton area, take Route 78 west to Exit 11. Cross over Route 78, following the signs for Pattenburg. Immediately after crossing Route 78, turn left at the light. Proceed to the remains of the stone Baptist church and bear right onto Baptist Church Road. Proceed on Baptist Church Road under a railroad bridge and, shortly thereafter, turn left into the park entrance, marked by a brown Hunterdon County Parks System sign.

For a cool walk on a hot summer's day, try Hoffman Park on Baptist Church Road in Union Township. Although not specifically marked, the trails are wide, following old farm roads and mowed paths, so ticks are a minimal worry. You can make it quick, say thirty minutes to one hour, or spend a half day.

This excursion is suitable for the whole family. Bring a stroller or a child's bike if you like, but be aware that there are hills. Perhaps your kids would enjoy fishing. If so, choose from five ponds originally created in the 1940s for erosion control, crop irrigation, and cattle management.

Manny's Pond is the largest in the park and easily accessible. Enjoy wonderful views of the park's features, as well as Spruce Run Reservoir and distant hills. The crisp air and foliage make this a special treat in the Fall.

Hoffman Park is also a great spot for bird watching. It is probably best known for species that nest in grassland habitats, including bobolinks, eastern meadowlarks, grasshopper sparrows, and savannah sparrows. Spot bluebirds year round in the fields and wood ducks in the wooded habitat near ponds or streams.

Envision Mr. Hoffman, son of the founder of the Hoffman Beverage Co., managing this 354-acre farm in its heyday in the 1940s and 1950s, a slice of rural Hunterdon. An ongoing stream restoration project and newly mown trails evidence today's efforts to keep the site viable.

You will know you've almost arrived at your destination of Hoffman Park when you pass the Bethlehem Baptist Church ruins off of Route 78, originally the Easton Brunswick Turnpike. The church was built in 1838 on land donated by Aaron Van Syckel, Jr., and the congregation grew to 125 members by 1857. Baptisms were conducted in a nearby stream.

Around 1868, members began leaving the rural church in favor of churches closer to their homes in Hampton and Clinton. The church closed its doors in 1906, although it came alive briefly in the 1930s for a wedding ceremony between Alice Woodard and Alman Ford Dyce, both of New York with summer homes in Hunterdon County. We can only conjecture that the couple was charmed by the historic stone church and selected it as the site for exchanging their vows.

There is a well-maintained cemetery in the church yard, with the oldest grave being that of Catharine Updyke Van Syckel and dated 1837. There are 40 Van Syckel gravesites within the iron fence.

To control the deer population, hunting is allowed in the park with a special hunting license issued by the County Parks Department in addition to a New Jersey Division of Fish and Wildlife license. Seven permits are issued for the 125 huntable acres. No hunting is permitted on Sundays. For complete details, please see the Hunterdon County Department of Parks and Recreation website, www.co.hunterdon.nj.us.

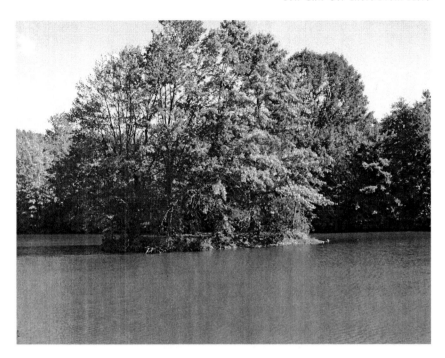

Hoffman Park - Manny's pond

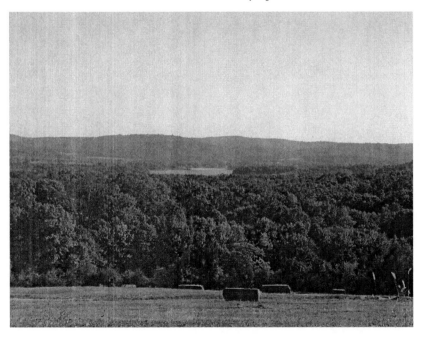

Hoffman Park - view of Round Valley

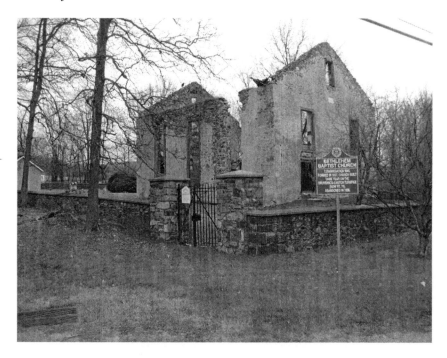

Hoffman Park - Baptist Church ruins

The Columbia Trail

Motivation is what gets you started. Habit is what keeps you going.
-- Jim Ryun

Difficulty Rating: Easy
Distance: 7+ miles
Sun/Shade: Shade
Location: High Bridge and Califon Boroughs, Clinton and Lebanon Townships, Morris County
Highlights: Views, gorge, dam
Restrooms: No
Parking: Gravel
Hunting: No
Directions:

> To park in High Bridge, from Route 31, go north on Route 513. Follow Route 513 into High Bridge. After about 1 mile and passing under the trail tracks, turn left into the center of High Bridge. Follow signs to the High Bridge Commons parking area on the left.

In the mid 1990s, the Columbia Gas Company constructed a gas line under the rail bed of the former rail line established by the Central Railroad of New Jersey in 1875. The surface rights were transferred to the Hunterdon County Parks Department for use as a recreational trail. The result is a wonderful, wide and mostly flat trail extending seven miles from High Bridge to the Morris County line.

Trail features include views of the South Branch of the Raritan River, a forest, and a diversity of wildlife. The trail passes through Ken Lockwood gorge. We recommend this trail for a family outing – walking, biking, or fishing – suited to whatever level of stamina describes your family. Cross-country skiing in winter is a bonus.

By all means check out the Califon station, now home to the Califon Historical Society. The station is open to visitors the 1st and 3rd Sunday of each month from May through October. Local residents have donated many items to the collection of memorabilia displayed by the Historical Society.

So you have reached Califon and still feeling fresh, it's a beautiful day and you have time, go on past the station and the Califon Lumber Yard where you will reach Vernoy Road. At that point, cross the road and continue the Columbia/Teetertown Trail in Morris County. Alternatively, you can follow the Columbia/Teetertown Connector Trail to the Teetertown Preserve. This is the kind of connection trail enthusiasts have looked forward to for a long time. There is now limited parking at the trail head on Vernoy Road.

There is no hunting allowed on this trail.

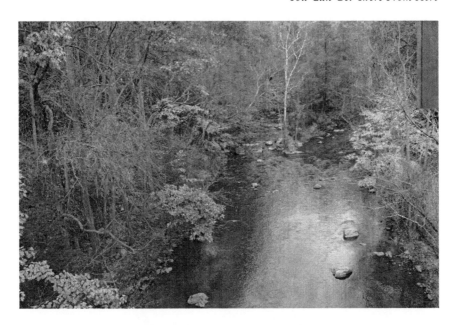

Columbia Trail - Ken Lockwood gorge

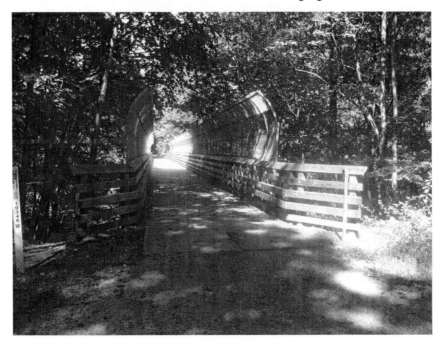

Columbia Trail - bridge over the gorge

Crystal Springs section of the Teetertown Preserve

One of the greatest principles of success – if you persist long enough you will win.
-- Og Mandino

Dificulty Rating: Easy to Moderate
Distance: 5 miles
Sun/Shade: Mostly sun
Location: Tewksbury Township
Highlights: Views, wildlife
Restrooms: No
Parking: Dirt
Hunting: Yes
Directions:

> Follow Route 513 north toward Califon. Just past the A&P, turn left on Sliker Road and proceed about 1.8 miles to Pleasant Grove Road. Turn right on Pleasant Grove Road. Look for a small green sign on the left that reads "47-51" and go to the end of that road. This is the park entrance. A grass parking area is on the right about 500 feet down the driveway.

Among the newest acquisitions of Hunterdon County and opened in 2008, Crystal Springs Park in Lebanon Township comprises 233 acres and offers something for everyone in the family. You may have to persist to find the entrance, but if you follow the directions specifically, you will be rewarded by locating this gem, which offers hiking, bird watching, and fishing. There are five ponds on the property, which are the headwaters of Spruce Run Creek.

Mineral springs found in the area are the source of the park's name. In 1815, the springs were found to be high in iron content and considered to be the purest source of water. The springs led to the creation of one of the earliest resort and spa communities in the country and is located on Schooley's Mountain in Washington Township, Morris County.

A walk through Crystal Springs is sunny, great for a chilly day, and long pants are recommended. From the parking area, turn right and follow the hedgerows and tree lines of former farm fields. The walk proceeds uphill from the parking area. Walk for a short distance or extend your walk by crossing into the next field. Do stay on the perimeter of the fields, which are actively farmed. Don't miss the views and do bring your binoculars if bird watching is of interest.

If fishing is your goal, cross the farm lane from the parking area and follow the trails to one of three fishing ponds. Each of these three ponds are designated for catch-and–release fishing. It is a short walk.

To control the deer population, hunting is permitted in the park with a special hunting license issued by the County Parks Department in addition to a New Jersey Division of Fish and Wildlife license. Eight permits are issued for the 247 huntable acres. No hunting is permitted on Sundays. For complete details, please see the Hunterdon County Department of Parks and Recreation Department website, www.co.hunterdon.nj.us.

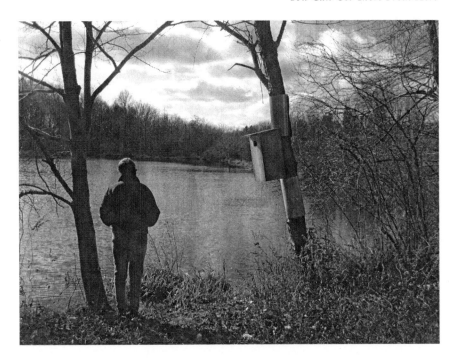

Crystal Springs - fishing pond

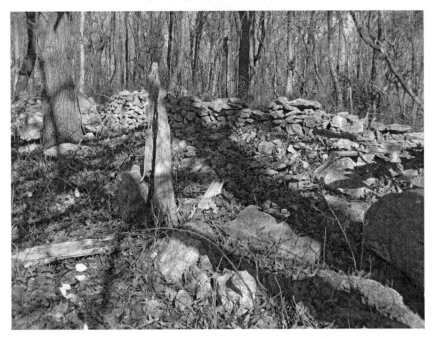

Crystal Springs - stonerow

Miquin Woods

The real secret of success is enthusiasm.
-- Walter Chrysler

Difficulty Rating: Easy to Moderate
Distance: 4.12 miles
Sun/Shade: Mostly shade
Location: Lebanon Township
Highlights: Woodlands, rocks, creek
Restrooms: No
Parking: Grass
Hunting: Yes
Directions:

> From the Clinton area, take Route 31 north to Glen
> Gardner. Turn right at the traffic light at Sanatorium Road
> and then left on Main Street. Proceed on Main Street and
> turn right on Hill Road (Route 628). Stay on Route 628
> about 3.5 miles and turn left onto Red Mill Road. In about
> 1.5 miles, turn right onto Newport Road. The park entrance
> is on the right.

Opened in 2008, Miquin Woods consists of 302 acres with woodland
trails first established in 1928 when the property operated as a Boy Scout
camp. For 53 years before closing in 1981, some 1300 scouts a year enjoyed
camping, fishing, nature, and crafts. Miquin means "feather" in Lenni
Lenape.

The trails are well marked and offer a nice variety of terrain and
opportunities for wildlife viewing. There is a great deal of shade, making it
ideal on a hot summer's day. Sturdy shoes and long pants are recommended,
and of course remember the insect repellent. Spruce Run Creek runs through

the park and feeds a small pond. We think this is an area suited to exploration by kids in the 8 to 12 age group – not too strenuous but challenging enough to hold their interest. It's also a peaceful walk in the woods if that is your motivation.

To control the deer population, hunting is permitted in the park with a special hunting license issued by the County Parks Department in addition to a New Jersey Division of Fish and Wildlife license. No hunting is permitted on Sundays. For complete details, please see the Hunterdon County Department of Parks and Recreation website, www.co.hunterdon.nj.us.

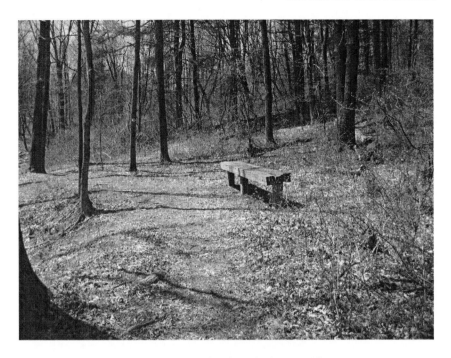

Miquin Woods - bench along trail

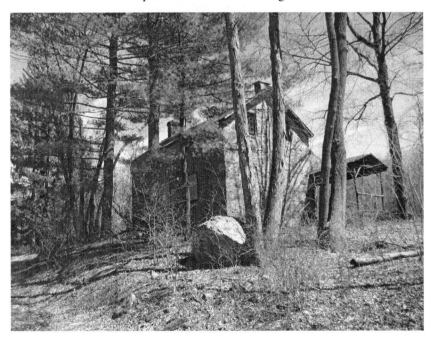

Miquin Woods - stone house

55

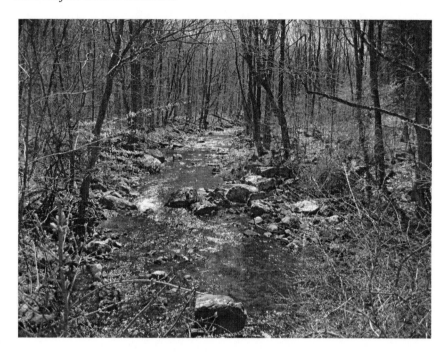

Miquin Woods - stream

Point Mountain

If you take the leap of faith, you will learn to fly.
-- Unknown

Difficulty Rating: Moderate to Challenging
Distance: 4 miles
Sun/Shade: Mostly shade, some sun
Location: Lebanon Township
Highlights: Scenic, rocks
Restrooms: No
Parking: Yes, dirt
Hunting: Yes, limited
Directions:

> From Route 78 in Clinton, take Route 31N (8 miles) to the traffic light at Asbury Anderson Road, which is Route 632. Turn right and proceed 4 miles to a stop sign at the junction at Route 57. Turn right on Route 57. At the first traffic light, turn right on Point Mountain Road. The parking area is on the left a short distance after crossing the bridge.

> There is also a parking area on Penwell Road. Follow the directions above, but instead of turning onto Point Mountain Road, proceed straight for 0.2 miles and turn right onto Penwell Road. The park entrance is the second driveway on the right after you cross a bridge. A small brown sign marks the sport. Taking two cars and parking one in each parking area, offers yet another option.

Part of the Musconetcong Mountain range, Point Mountain is the third highest point in the county. Four miles of trails through the 700 acres comprising the park can be described as arduous and scenic. Hiking boots are in order, and the overlook is a great place to stop, rest, take photos, and have a snack.

For a challenge, our recommendation is to tackle the steep, rocky "orange" trail from the parking lot on Point Mountain Road. After enjoying the overlook, continue on the orange trail until it intersects with the "blue" trail, which provides a lovely walk along the Musconetcong River.

Along the way, you may have the opportunity to observe more than 160 species of birds. The rocky terrain provides habitat for reptiles while the streams and river offer habitat for amphibians. And you may be treated to a sighting of more elusive mammals, including foxes, coyotes, and black bears. This hike could be a great adventure for families with children age 8 or 9 and older.

Fishing is also an option. If you have only one hour, park at Point Mountain Road and enjoy the river trail. Look up and see the wood duck nesting boxes that are protected from muskrat invasions by metal wrapped on the poles supporting the nesting boxes.

To control the deer population, hunting is allowed in the park with a special hunting license issued by the County Parks Department in addition to a New Jersey Division of Fish and Wildlife license. Twelve permits are issued for the 340 huntable acres. No hunting is permitted on Sundays. For complete details, please see the Hunterdon County Department of Parks and Recreation website, www.co.hunterdon.nj.us.

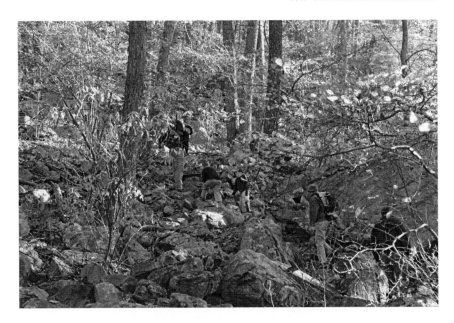

Point Mountain - the climb

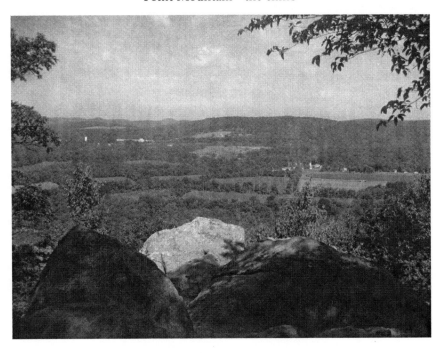

Point Mountain - Overlook

Teetertown Preserve and the Mountain Farm Section

To get what you've never had, you must do what you've never done.
Unknown

Difficulty Rating: Easy to Challenging
Distance: 5.4 miles
Sun/Shade: Mostly shade, some sun
Location: Lebanon Township
Highlights: Meadows, woods, habitat, water
Restrooms: Yes, portable restrooms at Mountain Farm
Parking: Yes, there are two parking areas for the Mountain Farm section and pull-offs for parking along Hollow Road
Hunting: Yes, limited
Directions:

> To Mountain Farm Section parking area: From Route 78 at Clinton, proceed north on Route 31 for 1.7 miles to Route 513 north. Turn right and follow Route 513 through High Bridge toward Califon for about 6.5 miles. Just past the A&P, turn left onto Sliker Road and proceed about 1.5 miles to Pleasant Grove Road. Turn right and travel another 0.6 miles to the driveway for Mountain Farm on the right-hand side.

> To Teetertown Ravine parking area: Follow the directions above except after 1.3 miles on Slicker Road, turn right onto Teetertown Road. Follow the left fork of the road approximately 1 mile to the stop sign at Hollow Brook

Road. Turn left and proceed 0.1 mile up the ravine. There are two single-vehicle pull-offs near the trailheads.

Established as the Lance family farm in 1749 by John Paul Lance, Teetertown Preserve/Mountain Farm/Crystal Springs today preserves 686 acres with multiple recreational uses. The Lance family constructed a farmhouse out of fieldstone in 1808. The home is still occupied today. The farm changed hands over the years and was acquired by Hunterdon County as open space in 1999.

This park area offers a variety of hiking terrain and features, including bird and wildlife sightings and interesting geology, making it a fun and educational family outing. Catch-and-release fishing is available in the two ponds at Mountain Farm. Also try your hand at native trout fishing in Hollow Brook. Remember your tick and bug repellant in summer.

Camping is available by reservation only.

For an overview of the park and about a one-hour hike, try hiking the Old Orchard Trail to the intersection with the Red Trail and head toward the ravine. Pick up the Geology Trail, which is steep, and follow it down to Teetertown Road. This is a dirt road with little traffic where you will get a great view of Hollow Brook, a spectacular rushing stream. Walk north on the road until you can access the Red and White Trail. Then turn north on the Red trail, which proceeds through a field and runs into the Pond Trail, which takes you back to the visitor parking lot. The hiking here ranges from moderate to challenging.

Shorter or longer options are available. After you get out there, the trails are well marked. There is a connector link starting on Hollow Road to the Columbia Trail. You pick up the connector trail where the Geology Trail comes out on Hollow Road, and it is 2+ miles to the Columbia Trail.

To control the deer population, hunting is allowed in the park with a special hunting license issued by the County Parks Department in addition to a New Jersey Division of Fish and Wildlife license. Fifteen permits are issued for the 298 huntable acres. Hunting is not permitted on weekends (5 p.m. on Friday to 5 a.m. on Monday). There is no hunting on Sundays. For complete details, please see the Hunterdon County Department of Parks and Recreation website, www.co.hunterdon.nj.us.

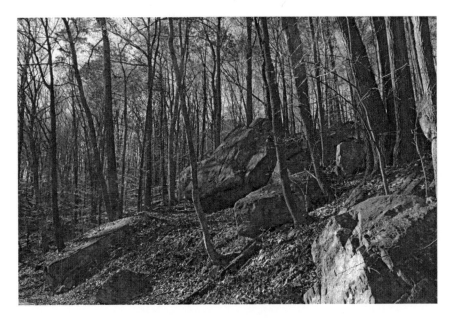

Teetertown - geology trail

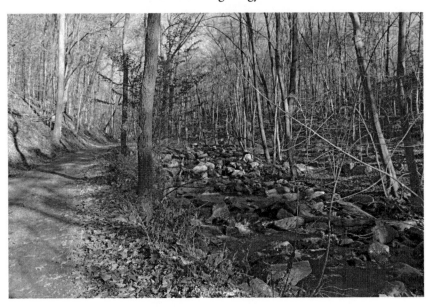

Teetertown - Hollow Brook

Voorhees State Park

You learn that if you sit down in the woods and wait, something happens.
-- Henry David Thoreau

Difficulty Rating: Easy to Moderate
Distance: 9 miles
Sun/Shade: Shade
Location: Lebanon Township
Highlights: Views, multi-use
Restrooms: Yes
Parking: Paved
Hunting: Yes
Directions:
> From I-78 West, take Exit 17, or if you are heading east take
> Exit 16. Then follow Route 31 North to Route 513 North.
> The Park is about 2 miles north of High Bridge.

Truly a multi-purpose recreational facility, the 1040-acre Voorhees State Park in Lebanon Township was developed as a result of the vision of Foster Voorhees, governor of New Jersey from 1899 to 1902. Once a farm with pasture, an orchard, woodlot, and farm buildings together with a home, Voorhees State Park was officially established in 1929, two years after Foster Voorhees donated his 323 acre farm, Hill Acres, to the state.

With the Great Depression engulfing the nation, President Franklin D. Roosevelt established the Civilian Conservation Corps (CCC) in 1933, which was a national job training program for single, unemployed young men. The CCC worked from 1933 to 1941 developing the park, including planting trees, constructing shelters and picnic sites, building roads and parking areas, and creating trails. The CCC work is at the heart of the facility that we enjoy today.

We absolutely recommend this park for the entire family. With trails, play areas, ball fields, picnic sites, camp sites and shelters, plus hunting and fishing, this park offers something for everyone. You and your family can spend many days exploring and enjoying this wonderful park.

Trails are well marked. Camping with reservations is available (tents, tent trailers, RVs, or 3 shelters), and restrooms with hot showers are nearby. Cross-country skiing is a possible winter outing. There is quite a nice park office, which is currently closed as a result of state budget cuts.

Try this moderate hike of about two hours. We recommend sturdy shoes and long pants. In summer, bug repellent will be welcome in your day pack, and do check for ticks at the end of your hike. Follow the Hill Acres Trail to the scenic overlook on Hill Acres Road. From this point, take in the view of Round Valley Reservoir. Continue on the Solar System Trail to the Paul Robinson Observatory, which was built by the New Jersey Astronomical Association in 1965. You may want to take advantage of their programs, which are offered year round.

Now go back to Hill Acres Road and continue to the Cross Park Trail, which takes you back toward the park entrance via Hoppock Grove. This walk through the woods and along Willoughby Brook gives a nice overview of what the park has to offer.

Are you drawn to water? Try the Brookside Trail that meanders along and over the Willoughby Creek, which runs year round. You can reach the Brookside Trail from the main road or from Picnic Areas A or B, which have their own parking or access via a short path behind the park headquarters building.

If fitness is your goal, try the one-mile 15-station parcourse near the entrance.

Hunting and fishing regulations are found at www.njfishandwildlife.com.

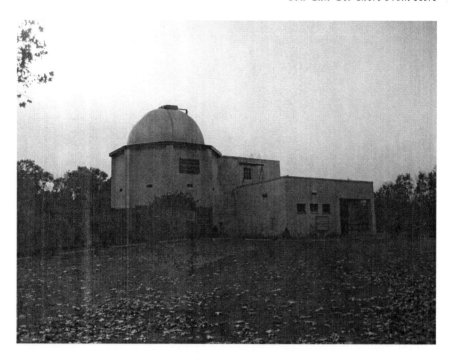

Voorhees - observatory

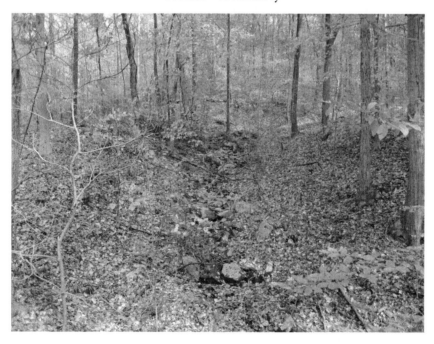

Voorhees - terrain

67

Cold Brook Reserve

Falling in love with the Earth is one of life's great adventures.
Steve Van Matre

Difficulty Rating: Easy
Distance: 2+ miles
Sun/Shade: Sun
Location: Tewksbury Township
Highlights: Views, wildlife
Restrooms: No
Parking: Gravel
Hunting: Yes, limited
Directions:
> Take Route 78 east from Clinton to Exit 24, Oldwick/ Whitehouse. Proceed north from this exit on Route 523 toward Oldwick. Continue straight on Route 517. After passing through the center of Oldwick, the park entrance will be on the left.

Sunny, rolling farm roads and fields characterize Cold Brook Preserve. This property consists of 287 acres, formerly a peach orchard and dairy farm. Beware of ticks and remember the bug spray. The walk is not difficult, and the opportunities to view raptors and discover habitats of small animals make this a great outing for families with children in the 8 to 12 range. Make sure that you have water before setting off on the 2+ miles of trails. Long pants are recommended.

When you are done walking, explore the Oldwick historic district, formerly called New Germantown. Stop in the Oldwick General Store, founded in 1750, for hot chocolate or lunch. Sit on the patio and have a drink at the Tewksbury Inn. Check out the treasures at the Magic Shop. This outing is a lovely way to spend an afternoon during any season.

Hunting is allowed in the park with a special hunting license issued by the County Parks Department in addition to a New Jersey Division of Fish and Wildlife license. Six permits are issued for the 179 huntable acres. No hunting is permitted on Sundays. For complete details, please see the Hunterdon County Department of Parks and Recreation website, www. co.hunterdon.nj.us.

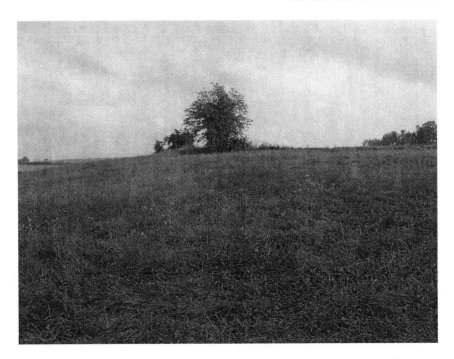

Cold Brook - meadows

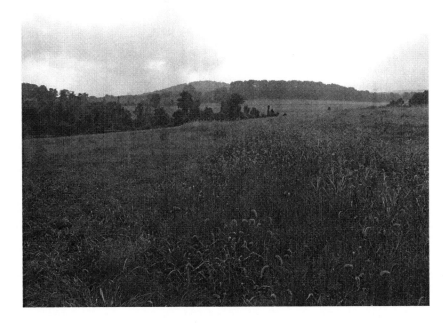

Cold Brook - distant views

End of the Trail

There is always another option to explore, another trail to tread.
-- Catherine Hartmann

This is just the beginning. We've shared a sampling of our favorite trails; Hunterdon boasts plenty more. We hope that you will get hooked on the beauty and the exploration while embracing the seasonal and developmental changes.

Thank goodness Hunterdon County is a community that treasures its open space, and the Hunterdon County Parks Department and New Jersey Division of Parks and Forestry do a great job on a limited budget keeping the trails user friendly.

Please do share your experiences on our website, http://www.get-there-from-here-books.com

Enjoy!

About the Authors

Alice Oldford lives in Hunterdon County with her husband, John. She is a Land Use Administrator, Realtor and freelance writer. She raised 5 children who grew up appreciating the joys of living in Hunterdon County.

Alice has been an avid walker since 1991, and her passion is enjoying the trails of Hunterdon County.

Sue Dziamara lives in Hunterdon County with her husband, John. She is a Professional Planner and earned her degree from Rutgers University .

She completed her first marathon in 1998 and continues to maintain her health through the exploration of Hunterdon County.

Breinigsville, PA USA
18 August 2009
222468BV00002B/2/P